THE EASIEST RECIPES ON EARTH

Cookbook

Enrique M. Joy

Contents

Chapter One

GRILLED PANINI

Grilled Panini with Goat Cheese and Fire-Roasted Pepper

It makes one sandwich.

Sandwiches can be both a godsend and a curse for people who are attempting to eat more healthily. When you order them at a café, you often have no idea how good the ingredients are or how much butter or fat is used to grill the sandwich.

So, instead of buying them, why not manufacture them yourself?

Here's a quick and easy way to prepare a delicious café-style sandwich.

2 slices of your favorite gluten-free multigrain or seeded bread

a few thawed frozen slices of grilled zucchini and eggplant (or make your own on the grill)

a sliver or two of delicious red or yellow pepper, fire-roasted (look for this in a jar near the pickles at the store)

1 ounce goat cheese (or a low-fat cheese of your choice)

to taste cracked pepper and sea salt or pink salt

Vegan spreads made with ghee, butter, or Earth Balance®

Add a couple slices of good-quality all-natural chicken or turkey for added protein.

On medium-high heat, heat a cast iron griddle skillet or a standard pan.

Use only a small bit of the butter you're using to coat the pan. Using all of the ingredients except the butter, assemble the sandwich. Place the sandwich on the griddle and use the bottom of another heavy skillet or a metal spatula to smash it down. When the edges of the sandwich start to brown, carefully flip it over and brown the other side.

Eat right away! Serve with a salad or sweet potato and beet chips for a healthy snack.

Chapter Two

MEXICAN WRAP

Mexican Wrap with Chicken and Chipotle Hummus for a Quick Lunch

Makes 2 or more servings

1 cup diced rotisserie chicken from the store

12 cup mayonnaise or Vegenaise®

1 chopped chipotle in adobo sauce (in a can, in the ethnic section of the store)

2 gluten-free tortillas (I prefer Gluten-Free Sandwich Pedals—Red Chimayo, but any gluten-free tortilla would do)

1 small shredded cabbage or slaw cabbage medley package (or about 2 cups shredded cabbage from the salad bar)

12 mango (diced)

14 cup coriander

slices of lime

12 cup red pepper hummus from the store (or plain hummus)

a sprinkling of pink salt

Dice store-bought rotisserie chicken and combine with Vegenaise® and half of the chipotle in a mixing bowl. To add spice and flavor, a bit of the sauce from the can can be added as needed. Toss in the shredded cabbage, chopped mango, cilantro, lime wedge squirts, and a pinch of salt. Stir gently, but not too much.

Combine the other half of the chipotle and the hummus in a small bowl. Make a thorough mix.

Using a gluten-free tortilla wrap, spread the ingredients on it. Place the chicken and slaw mixture on top. Serve open-faced or folded up with slices of avocado. If preferred, top with a squeeze of lime.

Chapter Three

CURRIED FLATBREAD

Curried Flatbread with Chicken and Hot Curry Paste for a Quick Lunch

Serve either hot or cold.

Makes 2 or more servings

1 cup diced rotisserie chicken from the store (or diced all natural chicken lunchmeat)

2 tbsp. Vegenaise®, mayonnaise, or nonfat Greek yogurt

14 cup coriander

4 teaspoons finely minced purple onion

1 small chopped ataulfo mango (or any other ripe mango)*

2 tortillas (gluten-free) (I like the Gluten-Free Sandwich Petals)

2–4 butter lettuce or romaine lettuce leaves

2–3 tablespoons curry paste (hot)**

12 chopped red bell pepper (optional)

If you have any leftover cooked sweet potatoes or yams, cube them up and add them to the chicken as well.

Place store-bought rotisserie chicken in a bowl with Vegenaise® and dice it.

Combine the eggplant relish and Vegenaise® in a medium mixing bowl. Stir in the cilantro, purple onion, and chicken gently but thoroughly. If preferred, add mango and a pinch of salt.

In a skillet, heat the tortilla wrap with a little cooking spray, ghee, or olive oil. On both sides, heat through.

Take each one off the fire and place it on a plate.

On the tortilla wrap, place a few lettuce leaves.

Place the curried chicken mixture on top of the lettuce in an equal layer.

Serve the sandwiches open-faced or wrapped up.

NOTE: Before adding the lettuce and chicken, brush a little amount of the Vegenaise® curry mixture over the cooked tortilla.

* If you can't get a ripe mango, don't bother—the frozen variety is bland.

** Look for Patak Binjal Eggplant Relish®, which may be found in the ethnic food department of most supermarkets. If you can't find it, use a mild curry paste or another hot sauce like harissa paste instead. Look for it in the refrigerator case with the hummus or in the shopping aisle with other Mediterranean dishes.

Chapter Four

PIZZA WITH CAULIFLOWER, TOMATOES AN PESTO

Pizza with Purple Cauliflower, Sundried Tomatoes, and Cilantro Pesto

2 personal-size 9-inch pizza crusts Preheat the oven to 425 degrees Fahrenheit.

Cauliflower comes in four colors: white, yellow, green, and purple, as well as three heirloom varieties: yellow, green, and purple. To me, they all taste roughly the same, but it's fascinating to experiment with the different colors to create new concoctions.

To make the crust:

4 cups purple cauliflower (or any other type), grated or finely chopped

1 lightly beaten big egg

114 cup part-skim mozzarella cheese, shredded

13 cup grated parmesan cheese (or pecorino romano)

12 teaspoon oregano, dried

chickpea flour, 4 tblsp (or other gluten-free flour)

a quarter teaspoon of garlic powder

To taste, a few dashes of pink salt and pepper

To make the toppings, combine the following ingredients in a large mixing bowl.

3–4 goat cheese medallions (more or less to taste)

1 cup sundried tomatoes (optional) (packed in olive oil)

12 cup olives (Kalamata)

12 teaspoon red pepper flakes, crushed

To make the Cilantro Pesto, combine all of the ingredients in a blender and puree until smooth.

Approximately 1 cup

1 cilantro bunch, entire

12 cup extra virgin olive oil

12 CUP WALNUTS OR PINE NUTS, LIGHTLY CRUMBLED

2 large garlic cloves, loosely chopped

1 lemon, whole and juiced

to flavor with pink salt and pepper

a pinch of cayenne pepper

On a rimmed baking sheet, place parchment paper.

Cauliflower, grated Cover roughly 2 cups of the crumbles with a paper towel in a large mixing basin. Microwave for 3 minutes with around 3 teaspoons of water. Cook for a few more minutes, or until the potatoes are tender. Remove from the oven and let aside to cool somewhat.

Combine the egg, mozzarella, and parmesan in a mixing bowl. Stir in the cauliflower, oregano, chickpea flour, garlic powder, salt, and pepper until everything is uniformly distributed. Divide the mixture in half on the parchment paper and flatten out to about 9-inch circles once it's been blended. If you don't have parchment paper, spray a baking sheet liberally with cooking spray before placing the cauliflower on it.

Cook for 10–12 minutes after topping the pizza crusts with goat cheese. The sundried tomatoes, Kalamata olives, and red pepper flakes are then added. Cook for a further 8–10 minutes, or until the crust edges begin to brown and the goat cheese begins to melt. Remove from the oven and sprinkle with cilantro pesto.

To make the pesto, combine the following ingredients.

In a food processor, combine all ingredients and pulse until smooth. Once the pizza is done, spoon it on top, or drizzle it on with a plastic squeeze bottle if you have one.

Chapter Five

PIZZA WITH TUNA AND ARTICHOKES

Pizza with tuna and lemony artichokes, capers, and Manchego cheese

This recipe makes two flatbread pizzas.

Preheat the oven to 375 degrees Fahrenheit.

1 jar marinated artichokes (9 ounces), drained and halved

4–6 tablespoons shredded manchego cheese or parmesan cheese

a pinch of red pepper flakes

2 garlic cloves, crushed and minced

2–3 lemon slices, juice

1 tsp olive oil (extra virgin)

2 tortilla wraps (gluten-free)

1 can Tongol Tuna, drained, packed with water or oil (or Tonnino tuna)

capers, 2–3 teaspoons

6–7 Castelvetrano olives, pitted and chopped (look for them on the salad bar—they're a vibrant greenish blue color)

a sprinkle of pink salt

peppercorns, freshly cracked

Top with microgreens or pea sprouts.

Optional: purple onion, finely sliced

To garnish, use fresh flat-leaf parsley, cilantro, or basil.

In a food processor, combine half of the jar of artichokes, the cheese, red chili flakes, garlic, and a pinch of pink salt and black pepper. Pulse until the mixture is just loosely combined. Pulse 2 or 3 more times with lemon juice and around 1 teaspoon extra virgin olive oil, then remove.

If using, place in a bowl with sliced onion. Taste and add extra lemon or salt if necessary.

Place two tortilla wraps on top of parchment paper on a baking pan that has been sprayed with cooking spray. Cover each tortilla with the artichoke filling. Overtop with crumbled tuna, capers, and olives. Top with any remaining artichokes.

Microgreens or other small chopped greens can be sprinkled on top after baking for 20–25 minutes.

Warm the dish before serving.

Chapter Six

WRAPPED SALAD

Wrapped Salad with Grapes and Walnuts in a Curried Sauce

This recipe makes 2–3 wraps.

Preheat the oven to 350 degrees Fahrenheit.

1 medium to large red yam or sweet potato, chopped with skins on

2 tsp olive oil (extra virgin)

to taste with pink salt

1 quinoa and brown rice packet, precooked (found in the grocery aisle)

2 tsp mild curry powder (or Patak's® Mild Curry Paste)

3–4 tablespoons mayonnaise or Vegenaise®

2–4 teaspoons Greek nonfat yogurt

12 diced granny smith apple (skins can stay on if desired)

12 cup chopped slivered almonds or walnuts

10 sliced and quartered red seedless grapes

2–3 tortilla wraps (gluten-free)

Fresh cilantro or thawed frozen peas are optional.

Toss the yam in a bowl with a thin coating of extra virgin olive oil. Season with a pinch of salt. Stir together and pour onto a parchment paper or tinfoil-lined baking sheet. Bake for 15–20 minutes, or until just tender, covered in tinfoil. Make sure they're not overcooked; they shouldn't be mushy.

While the yam is boiling, combine the precooked quinoa and brown rice mixture with the curry powder in the same bowl. If you're using Patak's Mild Curry Paste®, combine it with the Vegenaise® and nonfat Greek yogurt in a separate bowl before mixing it into the rice.

Gently whisk in the Vegenaise®, Greek yogurt, apple, almonds, and grapes to coat.

Remove the yams from the oven and set them aside to cool.

Toss them into the mixing dish with the other ingredients and toss to combine. Season with salt and pepper to taste. If preferred, add fresh cilantro and/or thawed frozen peas.

Place on tortillas and roll up to consume.

Other options: prepare a little extra sauce with the yogurt, curry paste, and Vegenaise® and serve a dollop on the side with each wrap for added moisture and flavor.

Red Pepper Hummus in a Quick Chicken Wrap

Serve chilled.

Makes 2 or more servings

2 tortilla wraps (gluten-free)

14 cup red pepper hummus from the store

1 julienne carrot (or shredded carrot from the salad bar)

3 tablespoons coarsely chopped purple onion

banana peppers, 3–4 teaspoons (from jar, diced)

5–8 slices all-natural chicken or turkey lunch meat (organic available from Applegate Farms®)

Sprouts of peas, broccoli, or any other vegetable

3–4 tablespoons mayonnaise or Vegenaise® (optional)

lettuce leaves of your choice (butter lettuce, romaine lettuce, etc.)

Blend a little harissa into the red pepper hummus for an extra spicy kick.

Place the tortilla wrap flat on a dish and evenly pour the red pepper hummus.

Combine the shredded carrot, purple onion, and banana peppers in a mixing bowl. Serve with chicken chunks on top. Add a dash of Vegenaise® or mayonnaise to the mix. Season with salt and pepper. Sprouts and lettuce should be added on top. Take a bite and wrap it up!

Chapter Seven

PIZZA WITH SHRIMP AND PEANUT SAUCE

Pizza with Shrimp and Peanut Sauce on Thai Flatbread

This recipe makes two flatbread pizzas.

Preheat the oven to 375 degrees Fahrenheit.

Serve with shredded cabbage slaw, rice vinegar, peanut sauce, and sliced peanuts on the side.

1 teaspoon extra virgin olive oil or toasted sesame seed oil

Approximately 4 tablespoons red bell peppers

a few purple onion slivers

8 precooked medium-large shrimp from the fish counter

Bragg's Liquid Aminos® (tastes like soy sauce but is gluten-free) 1–2 tablespoons

2 tortilla wraps (gluten-free)

San-J Thai Peanut Sauce® (gluten-free!) around 14 cup

2–3 tbsp. chopped toasted almonds, cashews, or peanuts

3–4 tablespoons finely chopped fresh cilantro

sesame seeds, 2–3 tablespoons

To make the Slaw:

2 cups red and white cabbage (mixed) or shredded cabbage package from the supermarket

Vegenaise® or mayonnaise (about 3 tablespoons)

cayenne pepper, a pinch

a sprinkling of pink salt

1 teaspoon rice vinegar or mirin, seasoned (either is fine)

3–4 teaspoons loosely chopped cilantro

To make the flatbread pizzas, combine the following ingredients in a large mixing bowl.

Heat sesame seed oil in a small skillet. Add the peppers and onion once it's really heated. Cook for 3 minutes, stirring frequently. Toss in the precooked shrimp and simmer with the Bragg's Liquid Aminos® for about a minute.

Remove the pan from the heat. Place two tortilla wraps on a baking tray lined with parchment paper. Distribute the peanut sauce evenly. Arrange the peppers and onions on each tortilla, then evenly distribute the shrimp.

Preheat the oven to 200°F and bake for 20–25 minutes. Peanuts, cilantro, and sesame seeds go on top.

Serve with a big helping of Asian slaw.

To make the Slaw:

Serve by combining all of the ingredients.

This recipe makes roughly 2 cups of slaw (enough for 2 servings).

Chapter Eight

PIZZA WITH BUFFALO

Pizza with Buffalo Chicken Flatbread

This recipe makes two personal-sized pizzas.

Preheat the oven to 375 degrees Fahrenheit.

The brand of ingredients you have on hand will affect the outcome of this recipe. Whatever the case may be, it's a delicious and quick lunch or supper option. This one will be a hit with the youngsters!

2 completely cooked chicken breasts

2 Sandwich Pedals® Chimayo Red Chile variety flatbreads (or any kind of gluten-free tortilla)

14 purple onion, cut into julienne

12 cup crumbled blue cheese or goat cheese

You like hot sauce from Louisiana or buffalo sauce from Buffalo (or a red bbq sauce)

a few cilantro sprigs, finely chopped

For the chicken, prepare the following:

Cut cooked chicken breasts into strips from the store or create your own: Using a little extra virgin olive oil, pink salt, and chipotle powder or mild chili powder, cover deboned, skinless chicken breasts. Spray a baking sheet with cooking spray and arrange the chicken on top.

Cook for 25 minutes, or until the internal temperature reaches 165°F. Slice into strips and set aside after cooked.

To make the pizza:

On a greased baking sheet, place flatbread or tortillas.

Bake for about 12 minutes, or until the onions begin to brown and the goat cheese begins to melt slightly, then top with chicken, onion, and goat cheese. Remove from oven and top with as much buffalo sauce as desired.

Serve immediately with a garnish of loosely chopped cilantro.

Chapter Nine

BACK RICED WRAP

Sumac-Herbed Black Rice Chicken Salad Wrap

It serves 2 people.

Serve at room temperature or chilled.

12 cup black rice (or a mixture of black and mahogany rice) (look for Lundberg Japonica)

1 cup veggie broth or water

4 oz. chopped rotisserie chicken or any fully cooked skinless and boneless chicken

lemon juice, 2 tablespoons

1 tbsp olive oil (extra virgin)

to flavor with pink salt and pepper

a quarter teaspoon of sumac

1 smashed and minced garlic clove

14 cup green onion, finely sliced

2 tablespoons flat-leaf parsley, finely chopped

2 teaspoons chopped cilantro

1 tablespoon chopped fresh mint

12 tbsp lemon zest

3 teaspoons chopped slivered almonds or pistachios

Optional: Before filling the tortilla with the salad, spread your favorite store-bought hummus on it.

Combine rice and water or broth in a small saucepan over high heat. Bring to a boil, then reduce to a low heat and cook for 30–45 minutes, or until the vegetables are soft.

If necessary, drain the extra water. Allow to cool completely uncovered.

In a large serving bowl, place the chicken. Combine the lemon juice, olive oil, salt, pepper, sumac, and garlic in a mixing bowl. Allow for a 5-minute rest period.

Gently whisk in the other ingredients, including the rice.

Serve open-faced or rolled up with the mixture on top of tortilla wraps.

Chapter Ten

MEDITERRANEAN WRAP

Open-Faced Mediterranean Wrap in a Hurry

It serves 4 people.

Pesto, feta, lemon, green or black olives, pine nuts, tomatoes, shredded rotisserie chicken, rainbow chard, and cucumber make a delicious wrap.

1 tsp olive oil (extra virgin)

12 cup roasted pine nuts

lemon juice (about 3 tablespoons)

1 teaspoon zest of lemon

3 tbsp. balsamic vinegar

1 tbsp olive oil (extra virgin)

1 garlic clove, smashed and minced

12 teaspoon oregano, dried (or half if fresh)

2–4 tablespoons minced flat-leaf parsley

2 cups completely cooked grains, chilled after cooking in water or broth

Grape tomatoes, Little Splendito®, or cherry tomatoes (about 112 cup)

2 cups completely cooked rotisserie chicken, diced (or any kind of skinless boneless chicken, diced)

12 cucumber slices, diced

12 cup pitted and chopped Kalamata olives

2–4 rainbow chard or kale leaves, deveined and sliced

14 cup chopped Peppadew red peppers (look for the roundish red peppers on salad bars)

14 cup feta cheese, crumbled

to taste with pink salt and freshly cracked pepper

2 wraps made from tortillas

Add roughly a teaspoon of extra virgin olive oil to a small skillet over medium heat. Stir in the pine nuts continually. Cook till golden brown, but don't overcook it. Season with a pinch of salt. If the pan becomes too hot to handle, lift it above the flame and whirl it around to circulate the pine nuts. Once golden brown, remove from the oven and set aside to cool.

To make the dressing, whisk together lemon juice, lemon zest, red wine vinegar, olive oil, garlic, oregano, and parsley in a large mixing bowl. Set aside with a pinch of pink salt and black pepper to taste. Allow 5 minutes for the diced chicken to marinade.

Gently combine all ingredients, except the tortilla wraps, in a large mixing bowl.

Season with salt and pepper to taste.

Fill a tortilla wrap with a large amount of filling and roll it up to eat. Alternatively, eat it without the wrap!

Seared Tuna with Edamame and Mung Bean Fettuccine with Peanut Sauce and Sugar Snap Peas is a quick and easy meal.

This recipe serves two people.

tuna steaks (one or two)

a few drops of roasted sesame seed oil

12 pound package (uncooked) Edamame & Mung Bean Fettuccine from Asian® Organic Edamame

1 cup snow peas or sugar snap peas

12 julienne sliced yellow bell pepper

12 julienne sliced red bell pepper

3 spring onions, chopped (along with roughly an inch of green stem)

Approximately 12 cup (or more) (gluten-free) San-J Thai Peanut Sauce®

Top with chopped cilantro, sesame seeds, or chopped toasted peanuts, if desired.

Allow tuna to rest at room temperature for 10 minutes before cooking.

Drizzle a little toasted sesame seed oil in the pan or straight on the tuna if grilling.

Sear tuna steaks on both sides in a skillet or grill, leaving the center pink if desired for medium rare, or until internal temperature reaches 125°F. If you want it more well done, cook it a little longer.

Allow time to rest when you've finished.

Bring 3 cups water to a boil in a medium pot. Toss in the fettuccine. Reduce heat to low and cook for 7–8 minutes, or until chicken is cooked through.

Drain in a colander and rinse with cold water when finished.

Add a bit more toasted sesame seed oil to the same skillet where the tuna was cooked. On high heat, add the vegetables and cook for 3–5 minutes, or until they begin to soften. Combine the noodles and the San-J Thai Peanut Sauce in a mixing bowl. Toss to coat, then divide between two plates.

Slice the tuna steaks into thin slices and arrange them on top of the noodles and vegetables. Add cilantro, sesame seeds, or chopped peanuts on the top.

Chapter Eleven

KABOCHA SQUASH

Roasted Kabocha Squash, Heirloom Spinach, and Sage Gnocchi

It serves 4 people.

Preheat the oven to 400 degrees Fahrenheit.

Kabocha squash is a pumpkin-like dark green squash with pale lines. When roasted, it has a very rich creamy sweet flavor—so sweet that you don't even need to add butter. It's delicious on its own, but it's much better in this recipe. When sugar pumpkins are in season, use them as an alternative. If you're in a hurry, precut butternut squash may be found in the vegetable department or frozen section of most supermarkets.

1 medium kabocha squash (or 1 precut butternut squash package*)

Extra virgin olive oil or a little cooking spray

1 package fresh gluten-free potato gnocchi (12 oz.)

Earth BalanceTM, ghee, or butter, 4 teaspoons

2 smashed and minced garlic cloves

nutmeg, a tiny pinch

8 large sliced fresh sage leaves, with a few more for garnish

14 cup broth (vegetable or chicken)

to flavor with pink salt and pepper

1 heritage spinach 6-ounce bag** (or regular baby spinach)

14 cup pepita seeds, raw or roasted

*This can be found in the produce section.

** Trader Joe's often has a fantastic deal on heritage red spinach!

For Kabocha Squash, follow these instructions:

Using a large chef's knife, carefully pierce the top of the squash and cut it in half. Remove the seeds and fibers before cutting the fruit into quarters. Place on a baking sheet and coat with cooking spray. Cook for about 20 minutes in a warm oven, or until just tender. When the skins are cold enough to handle, take them off with a paring knife and chop into 1-inch slices.

To make the gnocchi, combine the following ingredients in a large mixing bowl.

Cook store-bought gnocchi according to package directions. Some gnocchi is sold fresh in the refrigerator case; others are vacuum-packed and sold in the freezer case or grocery aisle.

Cook butter, garlic, nutmeg, sage, and vegetable broth in a large skillet over medium heat. Stir in the gnocchi, pink salt, and black pepper to combine. In a large mixing bowl, combine the squash and the entire bag of spinach. At first, this will be heaped over the skillet, but it will quickly wilt down into the skillet. To coat all of the ingredients, carefully whisk them together.

Toss in pepita seeds once the spinach has wilted. Season with salt and pepper to taste, and serve right away.

Chapter Twelve

SPAGHETTI

Spaghetti with Almond-Crusted Chicken and Adzuki Beans

It serves 2 people.

Preheat the oven to 425 degrees Fahrenheit.

34 cup almond flour

12 teaspoon parsley (dry)

14 teaspoon black pepper, roughly ground

a quarter teaspoon of salt

a pinch of cayenne

1 quart of yogurt

2 garlic cloves, crushed and minced

2 skinless, boneless chicken breasts

12 oz. adzuki bean pasta

1 12.5 oz. fire-roasted tomato can

4-5 Peppadew peppers, chopped (they're bright red and roundish and may be found on salad bars)

Garnish with flat-leaf parsley or basil.

In a small mixing dish, combine the first five ingredients.

In a mixing dish, combine the yogurt, garlic, and a few dashes of salt. Toss in the chicken to lightly coat it.

Place the chicken on an aluminum foil-lined baking sheet after dipping it in the seasoned almond mixture.

Add a bit more dry mixture to the top and pat it down onto the chicken.

Roast for 15–18 minutes, or until the internal temperature reaches 165°F.

Bring about 3 cups of water to a boil in a medium pot while the chicken is baking. Toss in the spaghetti. Reduce heat to low and cook for 7–8 minutes, or until chicken is cooked through.

Drain in a colander and rinse with cold water when finished.

Toss tomatoes and Peppadew peppers in a skillet. Cook until heated over medium-high heat. Toss in the noodles and toss to coat. Cook for a another minute or two.

Serve on a platter with the chicken on top.

If desired, garnish with chopped flat-leaf parsley or basil.

Chapter Thirteen

POLENTA

Polenta with Green Chili and Cotija Cheese and Fire-Roasted Tomatoes

It serves 6 people.

To make the polenta, combine all of the ingredients in a large mixing bowl

6 pints water

2 polenta cups Polenta Mix by Bob's Red Mill

12 teaspoon salt (pink or sea)

3 tablespoons unsalted butter

1 teaspoon powdered chipotle

1 teaspoon powdered garlic

Cooking spray or extra virgin olive oil

To make the toppings, combine the following ingredients in a large mixing bowl.

1 drained 15-ounce can of fire-roasted tomatoes with green chiles

34 cup crumbled cotija cheese (or queso fresco)

Fresh cilantro and a sprinkle of chipotle powder are optional garnishes.

Bring water and salt to a boil in a big, deep pan over high heat. Slowly drizzle in the polenta, stirring constantly. Reduce heat to low and cook for 30 minutes, stirring periodically to avoid sticking. Use a long-handled spoon to stir the mixture since it will bubble up and burn your hand. Stir in the butter, chipotle powder, and garlic powder for a further minute.

Using cooking spray, lightly coat the interior of a deep, medium-sized bowl. Place the polenta mixture in the bowl and let aside for 10 minutes. Invert onto a flat plate once firm.

If you want to cut it into wedges and top it with toppings, it's ready to eat immediately. Cut polenta into wedge forms and place on a hot grill that has been sprayed with grilling spray if you want to add lovely grill marks. Cook for 3–5 minutes per side, covered, until lovely grill marks appear.

Place on a serving plate after removing from the grill. Add the fire-roasted tomatoes, cotija cheese crumbles, and cilantro to the top. Serve with a sprinkle of cilantro powder or mild chili powder on top.

Chapter Fourteen

PESTO MEATBALLS

Pesto Meatballs with Edamame Mung Bean Fettuccine

Serves 2–3 people

grass-fed ground beef, 1 pound

ketchup, 4 tblsp.

4 teaspoons finely minced onion

1 teaspoon powdered garlic

2 TBS WORCESTERSHIRE SEASONING

Black pepper and pink salt

a small amount of extra virgin olive oil

12 package Edamame Mung Bean Noodles® from Explore Asia

34 to 1 cup fresh pesto sauce from the store (look for it in the refrigerator case)

2 cups baby spinach (fresh)

6-10 half-sliced sundried tomatoes

3–4 teaspoons grated parmesan

2-3 tablespoons goat cheese, crumbled

Combine ground beef, ketchup, onion, garlic powder, Worcestershire sauce, salt, and pepper in a medium mixing bowl. Make little 1-inch meatballs from the mixture.

Heat a skillet with a drizzle of olive or grapeseed oil over medium-high heat.

When the pan is hot, add the meatballs and cook for 5–6 minutes, or until the internal temperature reaches 165 degrees F. Set aside once cooked.

Bring 3 cups water to a boil in a medium pot. Toss in the noodles. Reduce heat to low and cook for 7–8 minutes, or until chicken is cooked through.

Drain in a colander and rinse with cold water when finished.

Heat the pesto in a large skillet over medium heat. Toss in the spinach and cook for 2 minutes, or until it has wilted down into the skillet. Stir in the noodles, sundried tomatoes, and cheeses until the sauce and spinach are evenly distributed. Toss in the meatballs and toss to combine. Serve right away.

Chapter Fifteen

SOUP WITH MUSHROOMS AND RICE

Soup with mushrooms, carrots, and Bhutan Red Rice

Serves 4–5 people

In this recipe, you can use any type of mushroom you choose. Dried porcinis have a rich flavor that pairs well with a variety of other ingredients. Add a few dried or fresh morel mushrooms if you can find them cheaply—they're quite rich.

2 tbsp olive oil (extra virgin)

1 onion, yellow

4 diced carrots

1 cup red rice from Bhutan

4 c. vegetable stock

2 c. liquid

12 cup sherry for cooking

14 ounces reconstituted chanterelle mushrooms

2 oz. fresh sliced king oyster mushrooms

12 oz. reconstituted dry porcini mushrooms

8 oz. cremini mushrooms, fresh

Earth Balance®, ghee, or butter, 4 tblsp

3 garlic cloves, crushed and minced

1 leaf of bay

2 teaspoons minced fresh parsley

1 tablespoon fresh thyme (about 112 tablespoons dry thyme)

1 teaspoon rubbed sage (dry or fresh)

to flavor with pink salt and pepper

Option: Place the dry mushrooms in a microwave-safe basin with a little boiling water and cook for 2 minutes, covered. Allow to sit for about 15 minutes on the counter to reconstitute. Set aside the water to use as part of the soup's stock.

Heat a little extra virgin olive oil in a big pot. Toss in the onions and carrots. Cook for about 4 minutes, covered, after sautéing. Cook, stirring periodically, over medium heat with the remaining ingredients. Cook for approximately 20 minutes, or until the rice is tender.

If you want the soup to be thicker, blend about 1 cup of the ingredients in a food processor and add it back into the soup once it's cooked.

Optional: add around 14 cup red wine to the soup while it's simmering for an even richer flavor.

Penne with Peppers and Spicy Mexican Chicken

Makes enough for a large skillet—approximately 4 servings

Drizzle extra virgin olive oil or grapeseed oil on top.

1 small chopped yellow onion

3 big smashed and chopped garlic cloves

12 julienne cut green bell pepper

12 julienne cut red bell pepper

12 julienne cut yellow bell pepper

12 julienne sliced orange bell pepper (or use more peppers if desired)

2 adobo chipotle peppers, minced (look for them canned at the supermarket)*

1 teaspoon dried or fresh Mexican oregano, rubbed

2–3 teaspoons chopped fresh cilantro

1 drained 12-ounce can of fire-roasted tomatoes with green chilies (or look for them in garlic too)

1 cup broth (vegetable or chicken)

8 oz. penne pasta (gluten-free)

2–3 cutlets of chicken breast, sliced into 4–6 pieces

to taste with pink salt and cayenne pepper

Serve with lime wedges, cotija cheese, and chopped cilantro on top.

*Alternatively, 112 tablespoons chipotle powder

Add a little extra virgin olive oil to a skillet over medium-high heat. Cook for 5 minutes after adding the onion and garlic. Cook for another 5 minutes, or until peppers are soft. 1 chipotle, oregano, cilantro, tomatoes, and broth, minced Season to taste with salt and pepper. Cook, stirring periodically, for about 5 minutes.

Cook the pasta as directed on the packet. After that, drain.

Add the spaghetti to the vegetables in the skillet and gently mix to incorporate. Then, while the chicken is cooking, cover and turn off the heat.

For the chicken, prepare the following:

Combine the chicken, a minced chipotle, and a pinch of adobo seasoning from the can in a mixing bowl. Add a pinch of salt to taste. Grill on a cooking spray-coated indoor grill top or a cooking spray-coated outdoor grill grate. Cook for 4–5 minutes per side over medium-high heat, covered, or until internal temperature reaches 165 degrees F. Remove the item as soon as possible.

Place the spaghetti and peppers on a plate and top with the chicken. Serve with lime wedges, cotija cheese, and fresh cilantro on top.

Chapter Sixteen

EASY PEASY PAELLA

Serves 4–6 people (depending on how hungry your guests are)

1 quart of clam juice (or more if you want to use the whole jar)

12 cup broth (chicken or vegetable) (or water)

12 cup crimson rice from Bhutan

6 smashed and minced garlic cloves

12 cup chopped white onion

12 large delicious red bell peppers, thinly sliced

12 large yellow or orange bell peppers, thinly sliced

2 pinches saffron (about 12 teaspoon)

pepper cayenne

2–3 links of all-natural chicken andouille sausage (make sure they are gluten-free)

1 peeled and diced tomato

Shelled, washed, and deveined if preferred, 6–8 large shrimp (leave tails on)

1 cup peas (fresh or frozen)

4–5 washed and scrubbed fresh clams or mussels

To taste, season with sea salt or pink salt and freshly cracked pepper.

14 cup of water

Flat-leaf parsley, fresh

2 lemons, seeded and split into wedges

Add clam juice, stock, and rice to a large skillet or paella skillet over high heat. Bring to a boil, then lower to a low heat. Toss in the garlic, onions, and peppers. Stir. Saffron and a couple shakes of cayenne pepper are added. Cook until the rice is cooked, about 15 minutes.

Cook andouille sausage links in a separate skillet until browned.

Stir in the tomato and cooked sausage in the skillet. Cook for 5 minutes after adding the raw shrimp. Fresh or frozen peas, as well as clams or mussels, should be added. Add a few cranks of freshly ground salt to the mix. If it's getting too dry, add around 14 cup or 12 cup of water.

When the shrimp are firm and pink, and the clams and/or mussels have opened, the paella is ready. Remove skillet from heat and set aside for 5 minutes to cool. Toss in the parsley and lemon juice. Serve with more lemon wedges on the side.

Chapter Seventeen

VEGGIE STACK

Veggie Stack with Mexican Black Beans, Red Quinoa, and Brown Rice

It serves 2 people.

Do you want to amaze a guest with a delectable dish? Here's a quick and easy method to cook a delicious low-fat dish with a lot of flavor. This recipe will benefit from the use of a biscuit cutter or a cooking cylinder.

2 medium zucchini, cut to a thickness of about 1/8 inch

1 Muir Glen Organic Diced Fire Roasted Tomatoes with Green Chilies® 12-ounce can

a squirt of olive oil

1 Seeds of Change package Fully Cooked Quinoa and Brown Rice® (or 3 cups fully cooked brown rice and 1 cup cooked red quinoa if you can't get it)

1 can organic black beans, 12 oz., rinsed and drained

1 teaspoon fajita seasoning or taco seasoning

Add a few crumbled cotija cheese sprinkles as a finishing touch.

a few cilantro leaves

Zucchini Preparation:

Coat the sliced zucchini with olive oil cooking spray and cook until tender on a cast iron griddle. Alternatively, heat until soft in a normal skillet, stirring once or twice until gently browned. Set away once you've finished.

Getting the Sauce Ready:

Puree the tomato and chilies in a food processor. Heat in a saucepan until thoroughly heated.

Stack of Beans, Rice, and Quinoa:

Add a dab of olive oil to a skillet over medium heat. Heat the cooked quinoa, brown rice, and black beans in the package. Add the taco seasoning and mix well. Stir in a handful of cotija cheese crumbs. Set aside once the ingredients have heated through, around 2–3 minutes.

Assembly:

Place the cylinder in the plate's center. Fill the cylinder with the brown rice/quinoa/black bean mixture using a serving spoon. Pack it firmly with the back of the spoon until it reaches the required height of 112–2 inches. Then carefully raise up the cylinder to remove it. Arrange a couple zucchini slices on top of the stack. Spread a thin coating of sauce around the stack using a spoon. Cotija cheese should be strewn throughout the plate. Serve immediately with a few cilantro leaves as a garnish.

NOTE: A biscuit cutter or a round kitchen mold with two open ends is required.

Shortcuts:

In the freezer section, look for completely cooked grilled zucchini and eggplant. They're fantastic!

NOTE: Any leftover beans and rice combination can be used to make an open-faced burrito for lunch later in the week.

Chapter Eighteen

RUSTIC CHICKEN

Asparagus, Sun-Dried Tomatoes, and Mushrooms in a Rustic Chicken

Serves 4–5 people

2 tbsp olive oil (extra virgin)

smashed and minced 2–3 big garlic cloves

2 boneless, skinless chicken breasts, chopped into thin slices

To taste, freshly cracked black pepper

Brown rice spiral pasta (about 212 cups) (or another of your favorite gluten-free pastas)

4–6 sliced cremini mushrooms (or use porcini mushrooms for richer flavor)

2 cups spinach (fresh)

14 cup goat cheese (plain) (not herbed)

1 cup seasoned fire-roasted tomatoes (available at salad bars) or 1 cup rehydrated sun-dried tomatoes

14 cup whole Kalamata olives

3–4 asparagus stalks, completely cooked

Optional: a few pine nuts and red chili flakes

Tip for Preparation:

Add the garlic to the olive oil and lay it on the counter covered between 1 and 3 hours before you start cooking. This will release the garlic's peppery flavor into the oil, adding a fantastic layer of flavor to the dish.

Cook the chicken in a skillet with a drizzle of extra virgin olive oil over medium heat, tossing periodically. Add some freshly cracked pepper to the pot while it's cooking. Remove from heat and set aside once cooked through, about 5–8 minutes.

Bring water to a boil in a pot and cook the pasta according to package directions. Remove from heat, drain in a colander, and set aside once done.

Drizzle a little garlicky olive oil in the same skillet as the chicken and throw in the mushrooms, cooking for about 3 minutes. After that, toss in the spinach. The volume of the spinach will decrease as it heats up. After that, combine all of the additional ingredients in a large mixing bowl. The goat cheese will gently melt and form a light sauce. If it appears to be too dry at this point, drizzle in a little more olive oil and serve right away.

*A jar of sun-dried tomatoes with olive oil and herbs is available. That's alright; but, some kinds include a lot of sodium. It's possible that using a container of dried sun-dried tomatoes and soaking them in warm water to rehydrate them before using them in the recipe is a better option.

Crumble with pears and cranberries

1 pie pan (about 8–10 serves)

Preheat the oven to 350 degrees Fahrenheit.

Filling:

4 large peeled, cored, and thinly sliced pears (about 6 cups)

coconut sugar (three tablespoons)

a quarter-cup of lemon juice

1 teaspoon zest of lemon

1 teaspoon extract de vanille

2 tblsp arrowroot powder

1 teaspoon ginger powder

a pinch of cinnamon

nutmeg (1/4 teaspoon)

a third of a cup of dried cranberries

2 tbsp. Earth Balance®, ghee, or butter

Topping for Crumbles:

a quarter-cup of quick-cook oats

a pinch of cinnamon

12 teaspoon extract de vanille

a pinch of salt

a quarter cup of coconut flour

a third of a cup of coconut sugar

1 cup cold butter (or 12 cup butter plus 12 cup coconut oil)

Add a dollop of strained Labneh or nonfat vanilla yogurt to the top if desired.

In a medium mixing dish, combine all of the filling ingredients. Fill a buttered/greased pie pan with the filling.

In a medium mixing bowl, combine the crumble topping ingredients with an electric mixer. Do not overmix the ingredients.

Evenly distribute the crumble mixture over the filling.

Cook for 20–25 minutes, or until golden brown on top.

Warm the dish before serving.

Chapter Nineteen

FRUIT TART

Fruit Tart with a Gluten-Free Base

This recipe makes one 9-inch tart.

Preheat the oven to 350 degrees Fahrenheit.

Have you heard about Labneh before? It's a luxurious strained yogurt that's incredibly tasty! Lebanese cream cheese is another name for it. This is something you'll probably find in a health food or Middle Eastern supermarket store. However, because it's so dense, it's quite heavy in calories!

If you can't get Labneh, don't worry; you can use any plain nonfat Greek-style yogurt—Fage® (pronounced Fah-yay) is the thickest I've found.

I used forelle pears for this recipe, which are petite and stunning with their scarlet speckles and yellow skin. They have a deep, fragrant flavor and a subtle crispness to them. When they're in season, look for them! Any pear will work in this recipe, but if you see forelles, keep them in mind.

To make the crust:

1 huge egg (from a happy, free-range hen)

2 cups flour made from hazelnuts (or use 1 cup hazelnut flour and 1 cup almond meal)

1 tbsp tapioca starch (or more if it seems too crumbly)

12 tsp fine sea salt or fine pink salt

2 tbsp coconut oil, melted or liquid at room temperature

1 tablespoon softened or melted butter

To coat, add extra coconut oil or coconut oil cooking spray (and more to coat the pan)

For the Creamy Stuff, combine the following ingredients in a mixing bowl.

strained Labneh yogurt (about 8 ounces) (or plain nonfat Greek-style yogurt)

1 teaspoon extract de vanille

12 tbsp lemon zest

To make the icing:

You can eat whatever fruits and berries you like! (I used forelle pears, sliced kiwi, blueberries, and raspberries.)

apricot preserves (about 14 cup) (look for all natural without added sugar)

1–2 tbsp. of water

In a food processor, combine the crust ingredients and pulse until they form a ball.

Scrape the sides down and remove the dough with a spatula. Place it in the center of a 9-inch metal tart pan coated with coconut or other cooking oil. Spread the dough out in the pan, pressing it down with the back of a large spoon or your hands. To make the edges even, tamp them down.

Cook for 15–18 minutes, or until the edges are slightly browned, on the middle oven rack. Because oven temperatures vary slightly, keep an eye on it to prevent it from burning.

While the crust is baking, combine the Labneh or Greek-style yogurt, vanilla essence, and lemon zest in a small mixing dish. After that, put it aside.

Allow it cool before carefully removing the tart with a spatula and placing it on a big dish or tray.

Evenly spread the cream mixture across the tart.

Without becoming too fussy, cover the tart with the fruit in whichever way you please.

To make the apricot preserves more liquid, add 1–2 teaspoons of water and stir with a spoon. It will have apricot pieces, which is acceptable; but, if necessary, add a little more water to ensure that it can be drizzled well. Drizzle the preserve "glaze" over the tart with a spoon.

With a sharp knife, carefully cut the pieces into wedges for serving. Be cautious while picking up the crust with a spatula because it may be extremely crumbly.

If you don't have a tart pan, you may make this in a 9-inch pizza pan. In fact, using a pizza pan makes things easier because the heated crust can simply be slid out onto your serving tray.

Chapter Twenty

VEGAN BLUEBERRY

12–14 servings

Preheat the oven to 350 degrees Fahrenheit.

I couldn't decide on a name for these. They were supposed to be scones, but they turned out to be more moist than scones. They aren't really muffins, either. So, I've decided to go with Blueberry Betty's! They're a cross between a drop cookie and a muffin, basically. And all you really need to know is that they're worth a shot!

1 c. almond flour

12 CUP CULTURED COCONUT FLOUR

12 cup tapioca flour

1 teaspoon salt (pink)

xanthan gum (34 cup)

1 teaspoon bicarbonate of soda

2 tablespoons powdered baking soda

112 tblsp cinnamon

coconut oil (four tablespoons) (room temperature)

112 tbsp vanilla extract

a third of a cup of applesauce

honey (three tablespoons) (or blue agave nectar)

13 cup plus 3 tablespoons unsweetened almond milk

If fresh blueberries are available, use 34 to 1 cup (if not use frozen, slightly thawed)

1 tablespoon sugar made from coconut

Combine almond meal, coconut flour, tapioca starch, salt, xanthan gum, baking soda, baking powder, and cinnamon in a medium mixing bowl.

Incorporate all wet ingredients (excluding blueberries) in a small bowl and mix to combine.

Incorporate the wet and dry ingredients in a mixing bowl and stir to combine. Gently fold in the blueberries.

Drop dough (approximately 2 tablespoons of batter) onto a cookie sheet coated with parchment paper.

If preferred, top with a sprinkling of coconut sugar and a pinch of cinnamon.

Preheat oven to 200°F and bake for 20–25 minutes.

Chapter Twenty-one

OATMEAL BARS

Chia, Pepita, and Flax Seeds in Raspberry Oatmeal Bars

Makes approximately 18 bars

Preheat the oven to 350 degrees Fahrenheit.

1 cup flour made from teff

a quarter cup of amaranth flour (plus 1 tablespoon reserved)

1 cup sugar made from coconut

a quarter teaspoon of pink salt

12 tbsp baking soda

flax seed, 1 tablespoon (brown or golden)

chia seeds (2 tblsp.)

1 pound of butter (softened and cut into pieces)

1 12 cup oats

2 orange zests (approximately 112 tablespoons)

pepita seeds, 4 tblsp.

raspberry preserves, 7 tblsp (low sugar preferred)

Combine teff flour, amaranth flour, coconut sugar, salt, baking soda, flax seeds, chia seeds, and butter in a medium mixing bowl.

Combine all of the ingredients until a crumbly dough forms. Mix in the oats and orange zest until everything is well mixed.

Using cooking spray, coat a 9 x 13 glass pan. Using about a tablespoon of amaranth flour, coat the pan. Any surplus that may have accumulated in the pan should be discarded.

Using your hands, press half to two-thirds of the dough into the pan's bottom. Serve with raspberry preserves on top. Gently press down the remaining dough on top. Pepita seeds are sprinkled on top.

Preheat oven to 350°F and bake for 35–40 minutes. Before cutting into bars, allow it cool fully.

Chapter Twenty-two

PINEAPPLE AND COCONUT MUFFINS

Little buggers that are dense and wonderful!

12 giant muffins or 2 dozen standard size muffins

Preheat the oven to 350 degrees Fahrenheit.

434 cup almond flour (or meal)

12 TBS BAKE INGREDIENTS

12 tbsp baking soda

Cinnamon, 212 tblsp.

12 teaspoon ginger powder (or use fresh grated for extra peppery taste)

12 teaspoon ground nutmeg

2 cups canned pineapple, smashed (retain the juice)

12 c. honey

a third of a cup of coconut sugar

14 cup room temperature coconut oil

3 teaspoons extract de vanilla

12 CUP OF PINK PINEAPPLE JUICE (from the can)

12 cup chopped walnuts or macadamia nuts

3 lightly beaten eggs

1 cup unsweetened shredded or flaked coconut, plus a little extra for sprinkling

1 cup grated carrot (about 1 large carrot)

1 large orange, zest and juice (about 12 cup juice)

12 cup unsweetened evaporated fat-free milk or almond milk

Using a spoon, blend all ingredients in a large mixing basin until well combined. Dust a large muffin tin with almond meal or other gluten-free flour after spraying it with cooking or baking spray.

Fill each muffin hole with about two-thirds of a cup of batter.

Add a teaspoon of shredded or flakes coconut to each muffin (about 12 teaspoon).

Cook for 45–50 minutes, or until a toothpick inserted in the center comes out clean.

Brownies with a Kick

This recipe makes 15 2-inch square brownies.

2 cups Gluten-free Baking Powder® from Bob's Red Mill

34 cup cocoa powder (unsweetened)

1 teaspoon powdered baking soda

2 tsp. cinnamon (ground)

1 teaspoon ground cardamom

1 teaspoon sea salt, plus a little extra to sprinkle on top of the brownies

1 teaspoon ground guajillo pepper (or another medium-hot chili powder)

14 cup room temperature coconut oil (or slightly more)

12 cup melted butter or ghee

1 tbsp extract de vanille

13 cup almond milk or water

Combine all dry ingredients in a large mixing basin.

In a medium mixing basin, whisk together all of the wet ingredients until thoroughly combined.

Combine the wet and dry ingredients in a mixing bowl and whisk until smooth.

Using cooking spray, coat an 8 x 11.5 glass baking pan.

Preheat oven to 350°F and bake for 45–50 minutes. Add a pinch of pink salt or sea salt on the top.

Before cutting into squares, let the cake cool for at least 10 minutes.

Chapter Twenty-three

BANANA BREAD

Gluten-Free Macadamia Nut Banana Bread

One 9 x 5–inch loaf pan is required.

Preheat the oven to 350 degrees Fahrenheit.

Bananas, macadamia nuts, and cocoa nibs: what's not to like? Not a single thing! Use this as a starting point for endless permutations with a variety of nuts!

1 teaspoon vanilla extract

1 cup sugar made from coconut

4 tblsp. room temperature coconut oil

6 tablespoons unsweetened almond milk (or milk)

2 lightly beaten eggs

mashed bananas (three ripe bananas) (can be previously frozen, thawed also)

1 cup flour made from hazelnuts

1 cup flour made from sorghum

1 teaspoon bicarbonate of soda

12 to 34 tsp cinnamon

2/3 cup macadamia nuts (or slightly more), chopped coarsely

12 cup cocoa nibs or chocolate chips, semi-sweet

Combine vanilla, coconut sugar, coconut oil, almond milk, eggs, and bananas in a medium mixing bowl. Stir until everything is completely blended.

Combine hazelnut flour, sorghum flour, baking soda, cinnamon, macadamia nuts, and cocoa nibs in a large mixing basin.

Stir in the flour mixture until it is completely incorporated with the wet mixture.

Coat a loaf pan with nonstick cooking spray and dust with sorghum flour. Remove any extra flour. Bake for 55–60 minutes, or until a wooden skewer or knife inserted in the center comes out clean.

Chapter Twenty-four

CORN AND CHEESE ON MUFFINS

About a dozen servings

Preheat the oven to 350 degrees Fahrenheit.

2 to 3 tablespoons chopped shallots

12 cup seeded and chopped red bell pepper

1 pound cornmeal (corn flour)

1 quinoa flour cup (or sorghum flour)

1 tablespoon powdered baking soda

112 tablespoons salt (pink or sea)

cayenne pepper (1 teaspoon)

paprika, 112 tablespoons (or 1 teaspoon Hungarian hot paprika)

1 lightly beaten big egg

1 cup unsweetened almond milk plus 1 tablespoon

a third of a cup of coconut oil

12 cup baby spinach, coarsely chopped

3 tablespoons chopped fresh basil leaves

12 cup parmesan or pecorino romano cheese and 12 cup cheddar cheese (half cup for the batter and half cup for the muffin topping)

Sauté shallots and red pepper in a small skillet over medium heat for about 4 minutes, or until tender.

Combine all other ingredients in a medium mixing basin, saving 12 cup of cheese for the muffin tops.

Toss in the shallots and red pepper flakes. With a spoon, combine the ingredients.

Fill muffin tins two-thirds full with batter in lightly greased or lined muffin tins. Sprinkle with a little more cheese and bake for 12–15 minutes, or until a toothpick inserted in the center comes out clean.

Before serving, allow it cool fully.

Chapter Twenty-five

LEMON POPPY SEEDS MUFFINS

For this recipe, use tiny muffin tins with paper liners.

This recipe makes approximately 3 dozen small muffins.

Preheat the oven to 375 degrees Fahrenheit.

12 cup almond flour/meal

a third of a cup of yellow corn meal

a third of a cup of coconut sugar

1 tablespoon powdered baking soda

12 teaspoon sea salt or pink salt

1 tablespoon seeds of poppy

14 cup unsweetened almond milk (or any other milk)

2 big, lightly beaten eggs

13 cup melted ghee or butter

3 tbsp. coconut oil (at room temperature)

2 lemons, juice and zest (about 12 cup)

In a large mixing basin, combine the dry ingredients and toss until well combined.

Combine all wet ingredients in a medium mixing basin and toss until thoroughly combined.

Blend the wet and dry ingredients in a mixing bowl and stir well to combine.

Fill paper-lined mini muffin tins two-thirds full with batter.

Bake for 10 minutes, or until a toothpick inserted in the center comes out clean.

Chapter Twenty-six

GINGER AND CARDAMOM MUFFINS

Makes one 9 x 5 inch loaf pan with a height of around 2 inches

Preheat the oven to 350 degrees Fahrenheit.

2 tablespoons almond flour

12 teaspoon sea salt or pink salt

3 tablespoons ground cardamom

1 cup sugar made from coconut

12 cup room temperature coconut oil (or melted butter)

12 cup maple syrup or agave nectar (blue)

3 big room-temperature eggs

apple cider vinegar, 1 teaspoon

1 teaspoon extract (almond)

1 cup crystallized ginger pieces/chips

Slivered almonds for the topping of the bars are optional.

Lightly coat a loaf pan with cooking spray.

Make a small well in the center of the almond flour, pink salt, cardamom, and coconut sugar in a large mixing basin.

Combine coconut oil, maple syrup, eggs, vinegar, and almond extract in a large mixing bowl. Slowly pour the wet components into the dry ingredients' well. To blend, stir everything together. Stir in the ginger chips.

Pour the batter into the prepared pan and bake for 45–50 minutes, or until a toothpick inserted in the center comes out clean.

Allow about an hour of cooling time before icing. Cut into 12-inch bars once frosted. If you're stacking them in an airtight container, use parchment paper or wax paper between layers to keep them from sticking together.

Chapter Twenty-seven

ESPRESSO BROWNIES

Adapted from my awesome friend Kelli Felix's recipe!

This recipe makes 15 2-inch square brownies.

2 cups Gluten-Free 1 to 1 Baking Flour® from Bob's Red Mill

34 cup dark cocoa powder, unsweetened (or regular baking cocoa powder)

1 teaspoon powdered baking soda

1 teaspoon sea salt, plus a little extra to sprinkle on top of the brownies

2–4 tablespoons espresso powder

134 pound sugar

12 cup coffee plus 3 tablespoons (previously brewed and cold or room temperature)

1 cup vegetable oil (or 12 cup coconut oil plus 12 cup mashed avocado)

12 cup melted butter or ghee

vanilla extract (two teaspoons)

Combine all dry ingredients in a large mixing basin.

In a medium mixing basin, whisk together all of the wet ingredients until thoroughly combined.

Combine the wet and dry ingredients in a mixing bowl and whisk until smooth.

Using cooking spray, coat an 8 x 11.5 glass baking pan. Preheat oven to 350°F and bake for 45–50 minutes. Add a pinch of pink salt or sea salt on the top.

Before cutting into squares, let the cake cool for at least 10 minutes.

Cookies with dates and nuts

Simply simply, these are incredible. Goji berries or other varieties of nuts can be used for a unique twist.

This recipe makes about 26 2-inch cookies.

Preheat the oven to 375 degrees Fahrenheit.

1 beaten egg

1 teaspoon extract de vanille

2 tblsp Earth Balance® or softened butter

1 cup oats (quick-cook)

12 cup almond flour/meal

Bob's Gluten-Free Baking Mix®, 18 cup

12 cup tapioca starch

12 CUP COCONUT SUCTION

1 teaspoon powdered baking soda

18 teaspoon sea salt or pink salt

1 cup pitted and chopped Medjool dates (or any kind of date pieces)

12 cup slivered almonds (optional)

Use parchment paper to line a baking pan or cooking spray to grease a baking tray.

In a medium mixing bowl, whisk together the egg, vanilla, and Earth Balance® until smooth.

Except for the dates, combine the dry ingredients. Mix with a spoon until everything is well combined.

Combine the wet and dry ingredients in a mixing bowl and stir until thoroughly combined. Stir in the date pieces.

Spoon roughly 12 tablespoons of batter onto the baking sheet that has been prepared.

Bake for 7–9 minutes, or until golden brown around the edges.

Remove off baking tray and set aside to cool for a few minutes.

To prevent sticking, put parchment paper or wax paper between stacks of cookies in a container.

Chapter Twenty-eight

LEMON AND COCONUT CAKE

1 9-inch cake (about 8 little mini-loaf cakes)

Preheat the oven to 350 degrees Fahrenheit.

To Make the Cake:

1 teaspoon tartar sauce

4 huge, separated eggs (but keep both the yolks and the whites)

a quarter teaspoon of baking powder

14 cup sifted coconut flour

pink salt, a pinch

honey (three tablespoons)

4 tblsp. room temperature coconut oil

112 tbsp vanilla extract

4 tbsp lemon zest (freshly grated)

4 tbsp. freshly squeezed lemon juice

12 CUP COCONUT SUCTION

Paper made with parchment

Spray cake pans with nonstick cooking spray (I used coconut cooking spray). Then use parchment paper to line the bottom.

Combine the cream of tartar and egg whites in a large mixing bowl. Whip for a few minutes, or until stiff peaks form.

Combine baking powder, flour, coconut sugar, and salt in a mixing bowl.

In a medium mixing bowl, whisk together the egg yolks, honey, coconut oil, vanilla extract, lemon zest, and lemon juice. Combine all ingredients in a mixing bowl. Sift the baking powder and flour mixture into the egg yolk mixture until it is completely combined.

To lighten the mixture, fold in about a cup of the egg whites. Then fold in the remaining egg whites, making sure they're as light as possible.

Fill cake pans two-thirds full with batter. Bake for 18–20 minutes, or until a toothpick inserted in the center comes out clean. Make sure not to overcook these puppies!

Allow to cool for a few minutes on wire cooling racks. Then, to finish cooling the cakes, flip them over on the rack and remove the parchment.

After the cakes have completely cooled, spread the icing on top. Once frozen, store in the refrigerator.

To make the icing:

a quarter-cup of coconut oil

1 teaspoon honey or agave nectar

1 teaspoon freshly squeezed lemon juice

12 tbsp lemon zest, freshly grated

a sprinkle of pink salt

12 cup goat's milk cheese

1 cup coconut flakes (unsweetened) (or shredded coconut)

Except for the coconut flakes, whisk together all of the ingredients until frothy.

With a spatula, spread the frosting on the cooled cakes. On top, strew the coconut flakes.

Keep the frosted cake refrigerated.

In the refrigerator, the frosting will harden up again.

Chapter Twenty-nine

COCOA AND GOAT CHEESE BARS

Makes around 20–24 bars

Preheat the oven to 350 degrees Fahrenheit.

12 cup gluten-free all-purpose flour (I used Bob's Red Mill®)

12 cup flour made with hazelnuts

1 teaspoon bicarbonate of soda

4 tsp cinnamon powder

allspice (212 teaspoons)

nutmeg (12 teaspoon)

1 teaspoon salt (pink)

4 quail eggs

12 cup sugar made from coconut

agave nectar (23 cup)

coconut oil (three tablespoons)

12 CUP APRIL APPLESAUCE

1 pumpkin can (15.5 oz.)

vanilla extract, 4 tablespoons

4 teaspoons melted butter

a pinch of salt

3 tbsp cocoa nibs (or chocolate chips)

Combine flours, baking soda, cinnamon, allspice, nutmeg, and salt in a small mixing dish.

With an electric mixer, beat eggs, coconut sugar, agave nectar, coconut oil, applesauce, pumpkin, butter, and vanilla until well combined in a large mixing bowl.

Mix in the flour mixture until it is just blended.

Using cooking spray, coat an 11 x 15 glass pan. Pour the mixture in and use a spatula to smooth the top. 30–35 minutes in the oven Allow for at least an hour of cooling time.

Cut into squares or bars after coating with icing. Refrigerate any leftovers.

Frosting with goat cheese:

12 oz. goat cheese, unpasteurized

12 cup softened butter or Earth BalanceTM

12 cup room temperature coconut oil

agave nectar (12 cup)

vanilla extract (two teaspoons)

Combine all ingredients in a large mixing bowl using an electric mixer. Refrigerate the frosting before applying it on the bars to thicken it. Refrigerate the frosted bars in an airtight container.

Chapter Thirty

PEPPER CHOCOLATE BUNDT CAKE

For this recipe, you'll need a bundt pan.

Preheat the oven to 350 degrees Fahrenheit.

To Make the Cake:

1 cup flour made from amaranth

1 cup flour made from coconut

1 cup sugar made from coconut

cocoa powder (four tablespoons)

2 tsp cinnamon powder

12 tsp. xanthan gum

1 teaspoon bicarbonate of soda

2 tablespoons powdered baking soda

12 cup tapioca flour

pink salt, a pinch

12 CUP COCONUT OLIVE OIL

2 big whisked eggs

1 teaspoon vanilla extract

12 cup semi-sweet chocolate chips or cocoa nibs

1 cup tart dried cherries

Except for the cocoa nibs and dried cherries, whisk together all dry ingredients in a large mixing basin.

Combine the coconut oil, eggs, and vanilla essence in a mixing bowl. Whisk until the mixture is completely smooth. Combine the chocolate nibs and dried cherries in a mixing bowl. Pour the batter into a bundt pan that has been sprayed with cooking spray.

Bake for 1 hour, or until a wooden skewer or knife inserted in the center comes out clean. Allow 5 minutes for the cake to cool before turning it over onto a wire rack to remove it. Place the wire rack on top of the bundt cake pan once it has cooled; flip it over and take the pan off the wire rack. Allow to cool completely before glazing.

You might want to move the cake to a serving pan before coating it.

Drizzle the spicy sweet glaze all over the top of the cake, allowing it to drip down the edges.

To make the Spicy Sweet Frosting, combine the following ingredients in a mixing bowl.

1 cup vanilla nonfat yogurt

1 goat cheese cup

1 teaspoon vanilla extract

2 teaspoons agave nectar or honey

12 teaspoon powdered guajillo (or any kind of medium-hot chili powder)

In a small mixing dish, combine all of the ingredients. Pour generously over the cake and allow it drip down the sides. Before cutting and serving, chill the frosting to thicken it.

Keep the cake refrigerated.

Sunburst (Pattypan) Squash with Stuffed Sunburst (Pattypan) Squash, Red Curry Shrimp, and Kaiwa

It serves 6 people.

Preheat the oven to 400 degrees Fahrenheit.

In season, look for sunburst or Pattypan squash. If they aren't available, yellow squash split in half lengthwise can be used instead. Simply scrape out a small portion of the yellow squash before filling.

12 c. kaiwa

1 cup water or veggie broth

1 minced garlic clove, smashed

to taste with pink salt

2 tablespoons finely chopped onion

6 “pattypans” with sunbursts

2 teaspoons red curry paste (Thai)

14 to 12 cup coconut milk (light canned)

8–10 thoroughly cooked medium shrimp, chopped into bite-size portions

4 tablespoons chopped fresh cilantro

2 limes’ juice

In a small saucepan over high heat, cook the kaiwa in 1 cup water or vegetable broth. Add the onion, garlic, and a pinch of salt. Bring to a boil, then lower to a low heat. Cook for 15 minutes, or until all of the water has evaporated. Remove from heat and set aside for 5–7 minutes. When you notice a little white thread coming out of the grain, you know it’s time to harvest it.

Depending on the size of the squash, cut the tops off around 12 inches from the top. Scoop out the squash’s insides and place them in a medium mixing dish.

On a baking dish coated with tinfoil or parchment paper, place the squash and the tops. Bake for about 10 minutes, or until the potatoes are tender but not completely cooked.

Combine the red curry paste and coconut milk in a skillet. Cook over medium heat while whisking together the ingredients. Add the cooked shrimp, cilantro, and a pinch of salt to taste. After that, put it aside.

Toss the cooked rice into the skillet and swirl to combine.

After the squash has finished cooking, stuff it with the kaiwa and shrimp mixture.

Bake for 15 minutes or until the squash is soft on a baking sheet. Remove the squash from the oven and pour fresh lime juice into the cup before placing the top on top.

Serve the squash with a wedge of lime and a sprinkle of chopped red pepper and/or fresh cilantro on top of the plate. Alternatively, sriracha sauce dots or zigzags can be used to embellish the plate.

Chapter Thirty-one

SALMON CROSTINI

Crostini with hot smoked salmon, hummus, dill, and capers

Makes 8–10 servings

Preheat the oven to 400 degrees Fahrenheit.

The measurements in this recipe are approximate because how you put the ingredients together is up to you.

4–5 slices gluten-free whole-grain bread

Cooking spray or extra virgin olive oil

a pinch of pink salt and a sprinkling of freshly cracked pepper

lemon juice (optional)

a quarter cup of chopped fresh dill

Per piece of bread, 112 tablespoons hummus

Capers (1/4 tsp) per crostini

Approximately 3 oz. hot smoked salmon

For each crostini, a pinch of hot paprika or smoked paprika

Remove the crusts from the gluten-free bread pieces and either give them to the birds or throw them away. Using a sharp knife, cut the slices into quarters. Brush each piece with olive oil and season with salt and pepper. Place on a baking pan and bake for 4–5 minutes per side, or until golden brown.

Mix a little fresh lemon juice and a couple tablespoons of dill into your favorite store-bought hummus in a small bowl.

Each crostini toast should have roughly 112 tablespoons of hummus spread on it. A few capers should be sprinkled on each slice. To each slice, add a few crumbles of hot smoked salmon. Serve with a sprig of fresh dill on top. Serve with freshly cracked pepper and paprika.

Other options: If desired, you can stir the capers into the hummus. Instead of hot smoked salmon, try hot smoked white fish—or both!

Chapter Thirty-two

BLACK RICE AND GOAT CHEESE YAMS

Approximately 8–10 pieces

Preheat the oven to 400 degrees Fahrenheit.

1 cup water or veggie broth

12 cup rice (black) (also called Forbidden Rice or mahogany rice)

2 huge red yams, peeled and washed, sliced into 12- to 34-inch thick discs

Tofurkey® Vegetarian Chorizo Crumbles, or any other natural sausage

(12 cup) crumbled goat cheese

Garnish with fresh diced cilantro or flat-leaf parsley, if desired.

Bring vegetable broth to a boil in a saucepan over high heat. Drain black rice after rinsing it in cold water. Add the rice to the boiling water, cover, and cook for 20–25 minutes, or until soft. Set away once you've finished.

Coat the yams in extra virgin olive oil or cooking spray and place them on a baking tray. Cook for about 20 minutes, or until the vegetables are soft.

Heat the chorizo crumbles through in a small saucepan or microwave.

Remove the yams from the oven once they are thoroughly cooked and allow to cool slightly before proceeding.

Place a tablespoon in the middle of each yam slice. Add the chorizo crumbles and goat cheese on top. Serve immediately after garnishing with fresh herbs.

Chapter Thirty-three

CROSTINI WITH MANGO AND PORK

Depending on the size of the tenderloin, this recipe makes 10–12 pieces.

For the best flavor, marinate the pork tenderloin for at least 4 hours or overnight.

If you want the pork to have excellent char markings, you can cook it on your outside grill or on an indoor barbecue grate. If you don't have either, simply bake for about 20 minutes at 350 degrees F on a baking sheet. If you have a digital cooking thermometer, it will assist you avoid overcooking the meat in this dish.

garam masala (3 tblsp.)

2 garlic cloves, crushed and minced

apple cider vinegar, 3 tblsp

4 tbsp olive oil (extra virgin)

1 pound plain pork tenderloin, cut into 34- to 1-inch thick medallions (plus or less)

a sprinkling of pink salt

Major Grey's Hot Mango Chutney®, 1 jar

6 slices gluten-free bread (crust removed) cut into bite-size pieces

Garnish with fresh chopped cilantro and/or finely sliced red bell pepper.

Marinade Ingredients:

Combine garam masala, garlic, apple cider vinegar, olive oil, and salt in a medium mixing basin. Make a thorough mix. Place the pork medallions on top. Cover and marinate for at least 4 hours, or overnight if you want even more flavor.

Allow pork medallions to come to room temperature while the grill heats up before grilling. Preheat the grill on high with the lid closed if you're grilling outside. Cooking spray or cooking oil should be applied to the surface of the grill grate once it is hot. Place the pork medallions directly on the grill grate and cook for 3–4 minutes per side, or until the internal temperature reaches 140°F.

Add cooking spray to the grill grate if you're cooking them on the stovetop. Cook for 4–5 minutes per side on the grill, or until the internal temperature of the meat reaches 140 degrees F.

Place a pig medallion on each piece of bread once it has been baked. Serve immediately with a dusting of fresh diced cilantro or finely diced red bell pepper on top of approximately 12 to 34 teaspoon of chutney.

Chapter Thirty-four

HARISSA AND POLENTA WITH FETA

This recipe serves 8–10 people.

To make the polenta, combine all of the ingredients in a large mixing bowl

6 pints water

2 polenta cups Polenta Mix by Bob's Red Mill

3 tablespoons unsalted butter

1 teaspoon powdered chipotle

1 teaspoon powdered garlic

112 tablespoons salt (pink or sea)

Olive oil (extra virgin) or vegetable oil

Toothpicks

To make the toppings, combine the following ingredients in a large mixing bowl.

1 jar harissa, tiny (about 8 ounces)

5–6 slices all-natural turkey lunch meat (Applegate Farms® is my favorite)

a third of a cup of crumbled feta or cotija cheese

Fresh cilantro and a sprinkle of chipotle powder are optional garnishes.

Bring water and salt to a boil in a big, deep pan over high heat. Slowly drizzle in the polenta, stirring constantly. Reduce heat to low and cook for 30 minutes, stirring periodically to avoid sticking. Use a long-handled spoon to stir the mixture since it will bubble up and burn your hand. Stir in the butter, chipotle powder, garlic powder, and salt for another minute.

Coat the inside of a deep medium-sized basin with cooking spray. Place the polenta mixture in the bowl and let aside for 10 minutes. Invert onto a flat plate once firm.

If you want to cut it into wedges and top it with toppings, it's ready to eat immediately. Cut polenta into squares or rectangles and place on top of a warmed grill that has been treated with grilling spray if you want to broil it and get excellent grill marks. Cook for 3–5 minutes per side, covered, until lovely grill marks appear. No worries if you don't have a grill; simply cut them into squares and move on to the next step.

Allow for a brief cooling period for easier handling. On each piece of polenta, spread a small amount of harissa. Cut the turkey meat into small pieces and roll it up on top of the polenta, securing it with a toothpick. If preferred, top with crumbled feta or cotija cheese and fresh cilantro.

Chapter Thirty-five

FLATBREAD WITH PROSCIUTTO AND MANCHEGO

Each tortilla yields roughly 5 pieces.

This dish serves ten bite-sized portions.

These can be made ahead of time and enjoyed at room temperature.

Preheat the oven to 375 degrees Fahrenheit.

2–3 gluten-free tortilla wraps, cut into bite-size pieces (I recommend Gluten-free Pedals®)

If Asian pears are in season, use 2 of them. If not, any kind of pear, such as forelle, can suffice.

14 cup manchego cheese, thinly sliced or shredded using a cheese knife

Prosciutto, sliced into strips (about 4 pieces)

Glaze of balsamic vinegar (not balsamic vinegar)

Arrange the gluten-free tortillas on a baking sheet and bake for 7–10 minutes, or until crispy and firm.

Cut the Asian pears into thin slices once cored and sliced. Skins can be left on if desired.

Place the tortilla wraps on a serving platter once they're done. Serve with pears, manchego cheese, and a couple strips of prosciutto on top. Drizzle the balsamic glaze in a zigzag pattern over the entire area, including the tray.

Serve right away.

* Because forelle pears are smaller than regular pears, you'll need roughly 5 of them.

8–10 servings Pistachio-Crusted Shrimp with Black Mahogany Rice

Preheat the oven to 400 degrees Fahrenheit.

When I serve the shrimp on their own, I use the dressing as a dipping sauce. You may add it to the rice for more taste or serve it in a ramekin beside the rice and shrimp on the plate. Choose your favorite!

1 cup dark mahogany rice (Lotus Foods Forbidden Rice® is my favorite)

a couple rough-cut sprigs of fresh cilantro

2 peeled and diced ataulfo mangoes (if not in season, look for regular ripe mangoes)

to taste with pink salt

1 cup roasted, salted, and ground pistachios

10 large raw shrimp, deveined and shelled; tails can be removed if desired.

112 egg whites with an ice cube whisked

To make the dressing (or use as a dipping sauce), combine the following ingredients in a mixing bowl.

1 cup rice vinegar (seasoned)

coconut sugar, 5 teaspoons

1 tablespoon red chili flakes, chopped fresh red fresno pepper, or seeded and minced red jalapeo

For the rice, follow these instructions:

In a large saucepan, bring the rice and 134 cups water to a boil. Season with a pinch of salt. Cover, decrease heat to low, and cook for about 25 minutes, or until all liquid has been absorbed and rice is soft. Remove pan from heat and let aside for 15 minutes, covered.

Place cilantro, 4 tablespoons dressing, and mango pieces in a medium-sized mixing bowl after somewhat cooled. Season with a pinch of pink salt.

For the Shrimp, prepare the following:

Pistachios should be ground in a food processor and placed on a platter. After the shrimp have been deveined and the shells have been removed, rinse them thoroughly and pat them dry with a paper towel.

Egg whites should be whisked together. Dip a shrimp into the egg whites and serve. Sprinkle the ground pistachio over the prawns with your other hand (rather than dipping into the pistachio). If you have it, place on a baking tray coated with parchment paper. If you don't have any, spray the baking tray with cooking spray. Place the shrimp in the oven once they are completely covered in pistachio. Cook for 7 minutes, or until the mixture is firm and opaque.

To make the dressing (or dipping sauce), combine the following ingredients in a mixing bowl.

In a small saucepan over medium heat, warm the rice vinegar. Stir in the coconut sugar until it is completely dissolved. Red chili flakes should be added at this point.

Placing the Dish on the Plate:

On each plate, pour roughly a quarter cup of rice. Serve with a shrimp on top. Drizzle some of the dressing over the shrimp and rice before serving. Garnish with chopped cilantro or minced red or yellow pepper.

Chapter Thirty-six

MUSHROOMS STUFFED WITH QUINOA AND RICE

This recipe makes 12–15 mushroom caps.

Preheat the oven to 400 degrees Fahrenheit.

Have you heard that your girlfriend is bringing a bottle of wine over? This one, on the other hand, can be made in a flash! There's no need to chop!

12 cup pitted and sliced date chunks or dates

3 oz. goat cheese with herbs

1 8.5-ounce package (Seeds of Change®) completely cooked quinoa and brown rice with garlic

12–15 cremini mushroom tops (about 112 inch wide)

cayenne pepper (a dash or two) or freshly cracked pepper

Garnish with fresh chopped chives or flat-leaf parsley, if desired.

Combine dates and herbed goat cheese in a medium mixing bowl. Mix in the fully cooked oats thoroughly.

Remove the mushroom cap's stalk and discard it. Pack the grain and cheese mixture onto the mushroom cap where the stem was with a spoon.

Place the mushrooms, stuffing side up, on a baking tray lined with parchment paper. Preheat oven to 350°F and bake for 15 minutes. Place on a serving tray. Fresh chopped herbs can be sprinkled over the tray if desired. Top with a dash of cayenne or freshly cracked pepper. Serve right away.

* If you can't find this fully cooked product, seek for other fully cooked gluten-free rices and quinoas in your grocery store. There's a lot on the market right now! Alternatively, you can prepare any gluten-free grain you want—about 2 cups cooked.

Chapter Thirty-seven

TOAST WITH KABOCHA

This recipe serves 10 people.

Preheat the oven to 450 degrees Fahrenheit.

1 212–3 pound kabocha, seeded and cut into 18–14-inch thick slices

a quarter cup of extra virgin olive oil

peppercorns, freshly cracked

12 tsp red chili powder

5 slices whole-grain gluten-free bread, split in half

Sea salt or pink salt

Garam masala, often known as hot curry powder, is a spicy curry powder.

5 grape or cherry tomatoes, half-sliced

chopped fresh flat-leaf parsley or cilantro

Slice the squash in half carefully by piercing the skin with a sharp knife. Cut the whole thing in half and then into four pieces. Using a spoon, scoop out the seeds and fibers and discard them. Coat the pieces with olive oil in a medium-sized mixing dish. Add red chili flakes and freshly cracked pepper to taste.

Place the squash on a baking sheet lined with parchment paper. Make a level surface.

15–18 minutes in the oven

Coat the bread with the remaining olive oil while the kabocha squash is cooking. Season with salt and pepper.

Place on a baking pan and bake for 4–5 minutes per side, or until golden brown.

Remove the squash from the oven and smash it lightly in a bowl.

On each toast, spread a spoonful of squash. Garam masala is sprinkled on top, and a tomato slice is placed on top. If desired, garnish tray with fresh herbs.

Chapter Thirty-eight

SNACKS FOR CHILDREN

212 cup rice (fluid)

1 cup potato flour

1 cup sorghum flour 1 cup sorghum flour

1 cup tapioca flour 1 cup tapioca flour 1 cup tapioca flour 1 cup tapioca

a quarter cup of cornstarch

14 cup garbanzo beans, soaked

xanthan gum (2 tblsp.)

Sift all of the ingredients into a mixing basin, then whisk them together with a wire whisk to ensure that they are well blended.

6 cup yield

Calories: 119; Total fat: 0.3 g; Saturated fat: 0 g; Cholesterol: 0 mg; Sodium: 1 mg; Carbohydrates: 27.2 g; Fiber: 1.4 g; Sugar: 0.1 g; Protein: 1.1 g

In a 14 cup fl our combination, there are 4.12 grams of fiber.

212 cup brown rice (fluid)

12 c. sorghum flour

1 cup potato flour

1 cup tapioca flour 1 cup tapioca flour 1 cup tapioca flour 1 cup tapioca

1 cup fl our coconut

a third of a cup of garbanzo bean flour

axseed meal, golden fl axseed

a quarter cup of cornstarch

xanthan gum (3 tablespoons)

Sift all of the ingredients into a mixing basin, then whisk them together with a wire whisk to ensure that they are well blended.

734 cup yield

Calories: 142; Total fat: 1.6 g; Saturated fat: 0.2 g; Cholesterol: 0 mg; Sodium: 1 mg; Carbohydrates: 29.1 g; Fiber: 4.12 g; Sugar:

0.08 g; Protein: 2.9 g; Carbohydrates: 29.1 g; Fiber: 4.12 g; Sugar: 0.08 g; Protein: 2.9 g

1

Snacks

Spread with a Spicy Cheesy Flavor

1 cup cheddar cheese, grated (Vegan Gourmet Cheddar Cheese Alternative is dairy-free)

2 tablespoons green chilies, chopped (canned) a quarter cup of mayonnaise

14 tsp. chili powder

Gluten-free tortilla chips (approximately 60 ounces) (Frito Lay Tostitos Bite Size Rounds Tortilla Chips are gluten-free) Q Preheat the oven to broil.

W Combine the shredded cheese, chilies, mayonnaise, and chili powder in a mixing bowl. Spread the cheese mixture over the tortilla chips using a knife.

E On a baking sheet, spread out the chips. 3 minutes in the broiler, or until the cheese is slightly browned.

Serves 20 (3-chip) people

One serving contains 41 calories, 2.4 grams of total fat, 0.3 grams of saturated fat, 0.7 milligrams of cholesterol, 72 milligrams of sodium, 4.4 grams of carbohydrate, 0.1

milligrams of fiber, 0.2 milligrams of sugar, and 0.7 milligrams of protein.

18

Taco Dip from Wheat-Free, Gluten-Free Cookbook for Kids and Busy Adults

12 tbsp. extra virgin olive oil

2 thinly sliced green onions

1 can (16 oz.) refried beans

14 cup of water

a quarter cup of salsa

a third of a cup of shredded cheddar cheese (Vegan Gourmet Cheddar Cheese Alternative is dairy-free)

Q Heat the oil in a small saucepan for 10 seconds.

W Over medium heat, softly sauté the green onions until they are tender.

E Add the refried beans and mix well. Cook, stirring regularly, until the beans are tender.

R Stir in the water until everything is well combined.

T Mix in the salsa until well combined.

Y Mix in the cheese until it is completely melted.

U Remove the dip from the pan and place it in a serving bowl. Serve with gluten-free tortilla chips as a dip.

12 (14-0 cup) serves

62 calories per serving; 2.6 g total fat; 0.4 g saturated fat; 1 mg cholesterol; 238 mg sodium; 7.3 g carbohydrates; 2 g fiber; 0.4 g sugar; 2.6 g protein Burger With Almost No Cheese

12 pound ground beef, lean

1 teaspoon onion flakes (dry)

1 pound cheddar cheese, shredded

(Vegan Gourmet Cheddar is a vegan cheese.)

Dairy-free Cheese Alternative)

14 cup milk (use casein-free soy or almond milk)

rice milk (for those on a dairy-free diet)

Snacks

19

ketchup (1 tblsp) (Heinz ketchup is gluten-free and dairy-free)
2 tablespoons mustard (yellow)

Q Coat a skillet in nonstick cooking spray. In a skillet over medium-high heat, brown the beef and onion flakes, breaking up the meat with a fork as it cooks.

W Reduce the heat to low and add the cheese, milk, ketchup, and mustard. Continue to whisk until the cheese has completely melted. Serve alongside gluten-free, dairy-free crackers or bread strips.

Serves 8 (12-cup) people

One serving has 123 calories, 4.8 grams of total fat, 1.2 grams of saturated fat, 33 milligrams of cholesterol, 257 milligrams of sodium, 6 grams of carbohydrates, 0.2 grams of fiber, 0.6 grams of sugar, and 13.5 grams of protein.

1 cup unsalted dry-roasted peanuts

1 tablespoon oil (peanut)

1 tablespoon of sugar

Q Blend the nuts together in a blender.

W Place the cover on the blender and pulse the nuts until they are finely ground.

E Blend in the oil, pausing regularly to scrape the sides of the blender with a rubber spatula.

R Blend in the sugar until the consistency resembles peanut butter.

Note: If you like your peanut butter crispy, add some finely chopped peanuts to it.

There are around 12 (1-tablespoon) servings in this recipe.

79 calories per serving; 7 g total fat; 1 g saturated fat; 0 mg cholesterol; 1.3 mg sodium; 3.5 g carbohydrates; 1 g fiber; 0.3 g sugar; 2 g protein

Chapter Thirty-nine

POPSICLES

cranberry juice (12 cup)

1 gallon of milk (use casein-free vanilla soy milk or sweetened almond milk for dairy-free diets)

3 teaspoons of sugar

Q Combine the juice, milk, and sugar in a medium mixing basin.

W Fill four Popsicle molds with the mixture, or use five-ounce paper cups.

E Freeze the molds for 4 hours or until they are completely frozen. When the liquid is partially frozen, insert a flat, wooden stick in the center of the mold, then freeze until solid.

Makes four popsicles

a single pop

77 calories; 0.04 g total fat; 0 g saturated fat; 3 mg cholesterol; 29 mg sodium; 16.2 g carbohydrates; 0.03 g fiber; 15.4 g sugar; 1.6 g protein

Drinks

Fizz of Lime

Combine different flavors of Coke and sorbet using your imagination. Try lemon sorbet with cherry soda or orange sorbet with orange soda.

34 cup Sprite (cold)

14 cup sorbet de lime (use dairy-free sorbet for a dairy-free diet) Q Half of the soda should be poured into a glass.

W Fill the glass halfway with sorbet.

E Pour in the last of the Sprite.

Serves 1 (1-cup) person

123 calories per serving Carbohydrates: 33 g; Fiber: 0 g; Sugar: 11 g; Protein: 0 g; Total fat: 0 g; Saturated fat: 0 g; Cholesterol: 0 mg; Sodium: 21 mg; Carbohydrates: 33 g; Fiber: 0 g; Sugar: 11 g; Protein: 0 g Lemon Mint Fizz

2 quarts of cold water

a third of a cup of freshly squeezed lemon juice (juice from 2 lemons)

Starters and Snacks

Mixed Spiced Nuts

6–8 people

Are you looking for something to eat as a snack? What about something you could serve at a party? Whatever your motivation, we're confident you'll enjoy these delightfully spiced mixed nuts at any time of day.

Ingredients:

a quarter-pound of butter

2 tblsp. salt, seasoned

1 teaspoon salt (garlic)

a pinch of cayenne

1 teaspoon of sugar

4 cups mixed nuts (pecans, cashews, almonds, walnuts, etc.)
Directions:

In the slow cooker, melt the butter.

Add the remainder of the ingredients to the slow cooker after it has melted. Cook for 30 minutes on high, covered.

Reduce the heat to low and continue to cook uncovered.

for

2

hours,

stirring

occasionally.

Before serving, remove the nuts and allow them to cool fully.

Per Serving Nutritional Information:

253 calories

17g total fat

339 mg sodium

Carbohydrates in total: 14g

8 g sugar

16 g protein

Chapter Forty

TASTY MEATBALLS

1 inch meatballs (about 24) Featured image courtesy of:

These are gluten-free thanks to soy milk and almond flour, but that doesn't mean they're bland. Serve alone or with your favorite sauce for a delicious gluten-free dinner.

Ingredients:

1 quart of soy milk

1 cup flour made from almonds

1 pound ground beef, lean

1 pound Italian sausage in bulk

1 pound lean pork ground

1 medium sliced onion

1/2 cup fresh parsley, chopped

three eggs

1 tsp. nutmeg

Ingredients:

Cooking spray, oil, or a slow cooker liner should all be used to coat the inside of your slow cooker pot.

In a large mixing bowl, combine the almond flour and soy milk and let aside to absorb the liquid. Combine the remaining ingredients in a mixing bowl. Mix everything together with your hands until it's just blended, being careful not to overmix.

Fill the slow cooker with your preferred sauce. Form the meat mixture into 1-inch meatballs using your hands or a scoop and place them in the saucepan. Cook for 1 hour on high, covered.

Reduce heat to low and simmer for another 3 hours, or until the meatballs reach a temperature of 165 degrees.

degrees

F

on

an

instant

read

thermometer.

Per Serving Nutritional Information:

123 calories

12 g total fat

245 mg sodium

Carbohydrates in total: 3 g

1 gram of sugar

15 g protein

Chapter Forty-one

CHICKEN WINGS

8 servings

Chicken wings are a simple source of entertainment.

meals, and using your slow cooker to prepare it frees you up to focus on more important tasks. For easy cleanup, serve these straight from the slow cooker.

Ingredients:

3 pound wings of chicken

1/4 cup extra virgin olive oil

paprika, 1 teaspoon

1 tablespoon honey

a half-cup of soy sauce

a half-cup of hoisin sauce

a quarter cup of rice wine

2 garlic cloves, finely chopped

1 teaspoon ginger paste (fresh)

Directions:

Cooking spray, oil, or a slow cooker liner should all be used to coat the inside of your slow cooker pot.

Preheat the broiler to high heat. In a large mixing bowl, combine the wings, oil, and paprika. Season with salt and pepper. Place them on a baking sheet and broil for 5 minutes.

minutes, until golden brown. Turn them over and broil for another 5 minutes on the other side.

Fill the slow cooker with the remaining ingredients. Toss in the wings to coat them.

Cook for around 3 hours, tossing once or twice to ensure that the wings are equally coated and cooked.

To keep things simple, serve straight from the slow cooker.

heated and drenched in sauce

Per Serving Nutritional Information:

476 calories

27g total fat

Sodium content: 501 mg

Carbohydrates in total: 16g

Sugars: 12g

Protein: 21g

CPSIA information can be obtained
at www.ICGtesting.com
Printed in the USA
LVHW060214160722
723616LV00015B/757

9 781804 769003